Protect Yourself fro
by l

CW00971766

Protect Yourself

FROM

Electromagnetic Pollution

BY USING

CRYSTALS

BARBARA NEWERLA

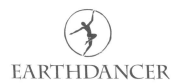

EARTHDANCER

A FINDHORN PRESS IMPRINT

Publisher's Note
The information in this volume has been compiled according to the best of our knowledge and belief, and the healing properties of the crystals have been tested many times over. However, bearing in mind that people react in different ways, neither the publisher nor the author can give guarantee for the effectiveness or safety of the use or application in individual cases. In cases of serious health problems, please consult your doctor or naturopath.

Barbara Newerla
Protect Yourself from Electromagnetic Pollution by Using Crystals

First edition 2010

This English edition © 2010 Earthdancer GmbH
English translation © 2010 Astrid Mick

Editing of the translated text by Claudine Eleanor Bloomfield

Originally published in German as
Heilsteine bei Elektrosmog – Was wirklich hilft und nützt
World Copyright © Neue Erde GmbH, Saarbrücken, 2009
Original German text copyright © Barbara Newerla 2009

Cover Photography: Ines Blersch
Cover Design: Dragon Design UK
Typesetting and Graphics: Dragon Design UK
Typeset in News Gothic

Printed and bound in China

ISBN 978-1-84409-509-4

Published by Earthdancer, an imprint of:
Findhorn Press, Delft Cottage, Dyke, Forres IV36 2TF, Scotland
www.earthdancerbooks.com, www.findhornpress.com

Contents

Foreword

The subject of radiation and electromagnetic pollution is more topical than ever before. The explosive proliferation of radio-technology for private use, particularly mobile phones, Wi-Fi and Bluetooth technologies, raises the question of the influence such developments may be having on humans and their health. All of these technological applications work with so-called 'pulsed high frequency radiation' and the effect on our health is a controversial issue, but some say the damage caused by this type of radiation could reach all the way to our genes.

This problem is actually not a recent occurrence. As early as the 1980s, when PCs began their triumphal march into offices everywhere and then later into our homes, many people became concerned about the stress caused by radiation given off by computer monitors.

In the early 1990s Michael Gienger, Anja Gienger and I founded our crystal wholesale trading company at the same time as increasing awareness of healing with crystals became known. It therefore seemed an obvious step to use crystals to protect against radiation from monitors. It quickly became apparent that certain crystals seemed particularly suitable for the purpose, and they are still considered to be the 'classic electromagnetic pollution crystals' today; however, new insights have since been gained in terms of how, why, and in what ways they work. And over time we have discovered that there are many more crystals that can help the human body cope with the burden of exposure to this kind of radiation.

Unfortunately there are also a lot of misunderstandings circulating regarding the use of crystals to protect against electromagnetic pollution. It is a matter of the greatest concern to me that this little book brings clarity to and sheds light on the possibilities, and also the limitations, of using crystals for this purpose.

What is Electromagnetic Pollution?

The term 'electromagnetic pollution' refers to the radiation given off by all man-made electrical, magnetic and electromagnetic 'fields' that surround us in our homes, offices and public spaces. We refer to something as being 'polluting' when we believe it to have detrimental effects on ourselves and/or our environment.

A 'field' is the space in which an electrical or magnetic force is active. In the case of an ordinary iron magnet, the field is, for example, the space in which the magnet is able to attract an object made of iron. In the case of an electrical or electromagnetic field, it is the space in which radiation can exert a measurable effect on an object or a body. The strength of the field decreases the further the object is from the source. In the same way, the damaging effects of electromagnetic pollution decrease the further away you are from the source.

These fields are created whenever an electrical appliance is in use or a transmitter is transmitting.

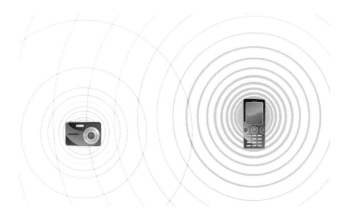

How and Where is Electromagnetic Pollution Created?

Electromagnetic pollution is present anywhere an electrical current is flowing. This means that there is electromagnetic pollution for a certain distance surrounding:

+ electrical apparatus or appliances
+ cables or leads of electrical appliances
+ electric cables in walls and in sockets
+ railway and tram lines

Electromagnetic pollution actually consists of two different types of field, magnetic and electrical:

The **magnetic field** is only present when a current is flowing, which means if an appliance is switched on or is in stand-by mode.

The **electrical field** may unfortunately also be present when an appliance is switched off, but when the plug is still inserted in the socket.

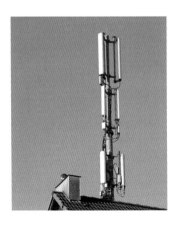

Electromagnetic pollution also occurs anywhere that radio waves are in use, for example the area surrounding transmitters. In such cases, electrical and magnetic fields always occur together, both types of field become indistinguishable, and the type of radiation emitted is called an **electromagnetic field**. Depending on the type and the strength, it may extend for several hundred metres to many kilometres from its source. Such sources include:

✦ radio and television transmitters
✦ mobile phone transmission masts
✦ radar transmitters (near military installations and air fields)
✦ cordless telephones
✦ access points for wireless computer networks and internet-connections (Wi-Fi); for example, in libraries, public places, companies, airports, railway stations, hotels
✦ Wi-Fi cards in laptop computers
✦ Wi-Fi routers in the home
✦ HomePlug
✦ wireless connections paired with various different apparatus (Bluetooth); for example, printer, keyboard, mouse, PC
✦ mobile phones

Does Electromagnetic Pollution Really Make You ill?

It has been stated, time and time again, that electromagnetic pollution and, in particular, the pulsed electromagnetic radiation of mobile phone traffic, has *no* damaging effects on the human body. This argument is based on the idea that the intensity of the radiation is far too low to create warming or overheating of the tissues. What is really being said, though, is that there is no visible damage, such as burns for example.

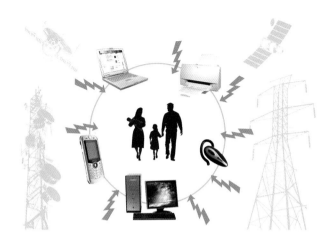

Unfortunately, no long-term research exists to prove that stress from electromagnetic pollution over periods of many years is safe. On the contrary, researchers are repeatedly finding indications that, despite the exposure being low intensity, the human body will be severely damaged in the long run. In addition, many people are discovering in everyday life that sooner or later they are suffering from problems that are unmistakeably connected with this kind of radiation, such as symptoms coinciding with the erection of a new mobile phone tower, for example, or the purchase of a new cordless phone.

Our own practical experiences as building biologists speak a clear message, as do the experiences of many sufferers, open-minded doctors, and therapists working in the field of natural healing: electromagnetic pollution (as well as other stress factors of modern life) causes massive stress to the human body; it facilitates and possibly triggers the rise of many illnesses, and even prevents a normal healing process.

The stress caused by electromagnetic radiation is referred to as 'electromagnetic stress'.

What are the effects of electromagnetic pollution? How does electromagnetic stress affect people? We will address these questions in the next chapter, and then go on to discuss crystals that may help.

Symptoms of Electromagnetic Stress

Often the initial symptoms of electromagnetic stress are relatively non-specific disturbances in a person's sense of wellbeing that cannot be connected with a specific diagnosis. This is what often makes the symptoms of electromagnetic stress so difficult to recognise.

A person might feel stressed, tired or exhausted, have headaches and/or circulatory problems, or be ill often. They may also have problems getting to sleep and sleeping through the night. Allergies may flare up or intensify.

The person may feel nervous and irritable, or even sad and depressed. Of course, all of these symptoms can be attributed to various

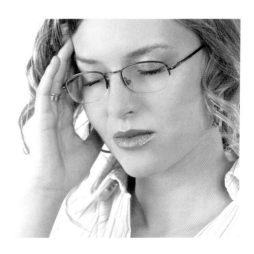

things, but very often stress from electromagnetic pollution lies at the root of the problem. Serious illnesses, such as cancer for example, or autoimmune diseases, may have electromagnetic pollution as a considerable contributing factor, but the disease may not develop until much later, or may develop as a result of multiple stress factors, including damaging environmental influences and psychological strain.

How do the Symptoms arise?

Electromagnetic pollution affects the body by placing it under continual stress! In addition to the other stress factors of modern everyday living, stress from radiation (such as from electromagnetic pollution) triggers a stress reaction in the human body, with all the associated short-term and long-term consequences. If we are subjected to radiation on a continual basis, the stress reaction is stimulated again and again. The stress condition becomes chronic, leading first to constant over-stimulation and finally to exhaustion within the organism.

How and Why Does a Stress Reaction Happen?

Over the course of human evolution, the body has adapted a pro-gramme that gets reflexively triggered in order to ensure survival when there is an acute threat. The body prepares itself for a fight or flight scenario. Hormones are released that make the heart beat faster, and the skin and internal organs are supplied with less blood in favour of a greater blood supply to the muscles and lungs. Blood sugar levels are raised in order to mobilise energy reserves, and thought processes are blocked in favour of programmed reflexive actions. This means that the capacity for logical thought and concentration are reduced.

Normally these hormones are dissolved and eliminated after the acute threat has passed, and the body is then able to regain its natural equilibrium. However, if the state of stress is maintained through constant stimulation, grave long-term consequences can develop.

Long-term or 'permanent' stress has become a serious problem in our modern western societies, so for many years now medical and psychological research has been looking into it.

The Consequences of Permanent Stress and Electromagnetic Stress

Stress Affects the Equilibrium of the Autonomic Nervous System

The autonomic nervous system controls all those 'automatic' functions of the body – the functions that are not influenced by the will. These include the activity of the heart, circulation, blood pressure, muscle tension, regulation of body temperature, digestion, and the activities of the internal organs. Also controlled by the autonomic nervous system are the sense of balance, the stress functions, the sleep-wake cycle and other rhythms that are related to time. Consequently, symptoms of a disturbance can be wide-ranging; every human being will react in their own way.

Symptoms of a disturbance of the autonomic nervous system may include:

✦ headaches
✦ digestive problems
✦ sleep disorders
✦ circulatory problems, high or low blood pressure
✦ heart rhythm disturbances

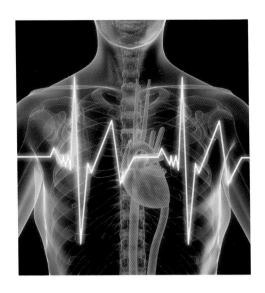

Stress disrupts the metabolism, provokes over-acidification and a build-up of toxins

Metabolic processes cannot function properly in a body under persistent stress. Persistent stress restricts blood flow to all the organs and tissues, and impedes normal functioning of the internal organs. The liver, stomach, intestines, pancreas and kidneys simply cannot work optimally, thus creating increased acidic metabolic waste products that cannot be eliminated effectively and are instead deposited in connective tissues. This, over time, creates over-acidification of the organism.

Over-acidification leads, for example, to tiredness and lack of energy, headaches, pain in the nerves and joints, tension in the muscles, and also encourages chronic inflammatory conditions.

Stress lowers the proper functioning of the immune system

During a stress reaction the immune system goes on the back burner, so to speak. If the stress remains unabated, for example because of the constant influence of electromagnetic pollution, there will be highly detrimental consequences in the immune response. Chronic stress causes decreased production of white blood corpuscles, and certain messenger substances are no longer secreted at all. This means you are more likely to become ill frequently, or succumb to an infection, and that infection is likely to heal more slowly or potentially turn chronic.

Stress has psychological effects

The fact that stress makes us nervous and irritable is well known. However, the latest research has also proven a connection between stress and depression. It has been known for a long time in the field of building biology that electromagnetic stress may trigger depression, especially stress due to high frequency radiation (mobile phones, radar, cordless telephones, Wi-Fi). It is also known that persistent stress, such as is caused by electromagnetic pollution, can influence the body's production of hormones. Where depression is concerned, the hormones

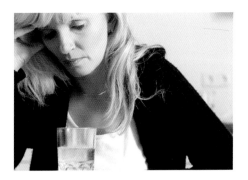

serotonin and dopamine play particularly important roles. When they are no longer produced in sufficient quantities, depression is triggered.

As we have seen, stress has far-reaching effects on physical and psychological equilibrium. If persistent stress continues over a long period of time, serious illness such as cancer or auto-immune disease may be the result.

How to Deal with Electromagnetic Pollution

In order for the application of crystals to bring real and lasting relief, it is imperative to reduce stress from radiation as much as possible; this is because crystals really *cannot* swallow or burn up radiation, or even shield you from it, though that is often claimed!

This goes for all appliances that work on modern radio transmission technology (mobile phones, cordless phones, Bluetooth devices, Wi-Fi), electrical appliances, and all electrical installations in the home and office.

You might also consider enlisting the help of a building biologist who specialises in the field of electromagnetic pollution as they can take measurements of the actual radiation stress levels and suggest ways to reduce or alleviate the problem.

How you can then use crystals for relief is described in the following chapters.

Crystals and Electromagnetic Pollution

In order to understand how crystals may help with stress caused by electromagnetic pollution, and also to identify what they *cannot* do, we need to distinguish between physical and energetic effects.

Physical Effects

An effect is *physical* when it is perceptible with our physical senses, or when it can be measured with measuring devices that work according to scientific physical principles. In the case of radiation this may mean that we are able to measure the strength of a field with a measuring device and produce results in a physically measured unit, for example in $\mu W/m^2$ or V/m. For cordless telephones, for example, it is possible to measure exactly how much radiation is affecting a person at a particular distance. If the apparatus is shielded with a suitable material, there is a clear difference in the measured values.

Energetic Effects

There are also types of radiation so subtle that they cannot be measured by means of the usual measuring devices. They are generally referred to as oscillations or vibrations.

This phenomenon is well known in terms of homeopathy, Bach flower remedies, and the application of crystals. As a rule, we refer to this effect as energetic rather than physical.

Objective and Individual Effects

As a rule, physical phenomena can be objectively perceived. This means that no matter who happens to be holding the measuring device, it will always register the same values. The effects may be perceived subjectively, but they can still be verified by different people. Anyone's finger will be burned if it touches a hot stove!

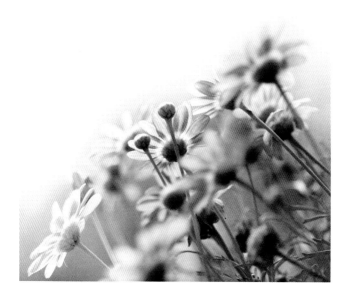

The more subtle an oscillation or vibration, the more individual will be the perceived effect. One reason for this is that energetic oscillations are mainly effective through what is known as 'resonance phenomena'. The strength of a stimulus may be very low, but if there exists within the person being treated a similar structure to the stimulus being given, the oscillation is amplified and takes effect because of the person's own reaction to it.

The Right Measures for Electromagnetic Pollution

Radiation and electromagnetic pollution initially have a physically measurable effect on the physical body, therefore physical measures are the place to start for protecting yourself from electronic pollution. You have to turn off the appliance, or find a way to shield* yourself from it. It is like you have to turn off the burner so that your fingers can't be burned. No crystal or other energetic measure will protect you from burns. You could use them later on to treat the burns and alleviate pain, but they are not a preventative measure. If you do not remove your fingers from the burner and do not switch off the stove you will continue to be burned, and even the most powerful energetic healing measures will not change this fact.

* There are many different possibilities for shielding against harmful fields, but please consult a professionally trained expert on the subject. (See contact addresses for building biology in the back of the book).

The Use of Crystals for Electromagnetic Pollution

Crystals can never replace building biological and physical measures, or a careful approach to radiation and modern technologies.

Crystals cannot shield us from electromagnetic pollution, nor make it disappear, as they do not work in a physical way, only in an energetic way. But they are able to support both our physical and our energetic bodies in dealing with the effects of electromagnetic pollution.

But again, they can only take optimal effect when we remove as many as possible of the 'coarse', interfering physical stimuli that block our ability to react and resonate with our own energetic systems.

Crystals can help us ...

✦ cope with the remaining inevitable stresses of modern life, as well as fortifying the body and the soul.

✦ alleviate or heal the consequences of previous stresses.

The effects of crystals target the places in the organism that were particularly affected and damaged by stress from electromagnetic pollution. There are a number of 'classic electromagnetic pollution crystals', and each will be discussed separately.

Notes on the descriptions of the effects of crystals in the following chapters
Many of the crystals described could be assigned to various chapters as they could be utilised in several areas relating to electromagnetic pollution. However, they will only be described in detail in chapters dealing with their main effects. Parentheses beside the crystal's name indicate certain keywords for the further range of effects, and correspond to individual chapters. For example, 'Agate' in the

chapter on 'Protection and Boundary Setting': **Agate** (→ Immune System, Stability)

At the end of every chapter you will also find a section entitled 'Additional crystals for...', which lists crystals that are described in another chapter but are nevertheless effective for the subject matter being discussed. The chapter in which the crystal is discussed in detail is indicated in semi-bold type.

For example, Garnet in the chapter on 'Regeneration': **Garnet** (→ **Strength and Vitality**, Immune System, Metabolism).

The Classic Electromagnetic Pollution Crystals

There are certain crystals most often associated with treating electronic pollution. Generally speaking, they are used for any type of disturbance, and often no distinction is made between radiation from the earth ('geopathic stress') and physical radiation from electromagnetic radiation. Especially concerning these 'classic electromagnetic pollution crystals' there is so much false information and stubbornly perpetuated myth, along with plenty of misunderstandings about their application.

Rock Crystal

When Rock Crystal was first used as protection against radiation from monitors, it was believed that the crystal would bundle the radiation and conduct it away. Larger or smaller pointed crystals were attached to the monitor so that the tips pointed away from the user. It is a fact that Rock Crystal points are able to conduct energy from their base towards the tip. With energetic treatments in particular, this property of bundling energy and conducting it away through the tip is utilised.

Light, too, is bundled and conducted within the crystal. Unfortunately the same does not occur with other types of radiation, including electrical and electro-magnetic radiation as emitted by monitors or other appliances. Rock Crystal cannot conduct the radiation away. If badly placed, Rock Crystal may even exacerbate the problem.

As Rock Crystal is inherently neutral it is very able to absorb information, store it and pass it on. That means, for example, a Rock Crystal that is placed on a 'disturbance' will in the worst case scenario even amplify negative oscillations and distribute them throughout an entire room. It will radiate these waves not only from its tip but also from its edges. The technically measurable, physical radiation will not change due to the crystal; there won't be more radiation or less radiation, so nothing really changes on that level. The energetic information coming from the disturbance can, however, become amplified under certain conditions and may negatively affect the climate of the entire room. *For this reason, Rock Crystal should never be placed on any disturbance spots, no matter what type, and the chosen position for the crystal should be tested with suitable means beforehand.*

If you wish to positively influence the climate of a room, place a Rock Crystal on a positive zone of the room so that it will radiate the zone's positive qualities.

The crystal may also be carried in the hand as a comforting object, or worn on the body, perhaps as a pendant. Since electromagnetic stress withdraws energy from the body, the properties of Rock Crystal may have a very positive effect. As a neutral energy supplier it has a fortifying effect on the body and spirit and can make you less susceptible to negative external influences. It improves perception, brings clarity, and makes you consciously aware. You may, therefore, be better able to recognise disturbances in your surroundings and have the means for removing them more quickly, before they are able to cause greater damage.

The application of special Rock Crystals may also be very helpful: The **Dow Crystal** balances energy lack and excess in the organism and strengthens self-organising abilities. **Faden** Quartz can strengthen your self-healing properties. **Channeling crystals** improve the ability of the body to perceive and realise its needs. **Accumulation crystals** have a building-up effect, helping to collect energy and help you to better manage your own energy supply. They help conduct away excess energy and clear the atmosphere of a room. **Tabular crystals** amplify all the body's energies and **Transmitter crystals** improve your communication with your body.

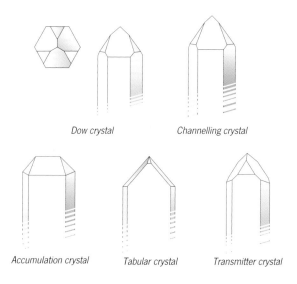

Dow crystal   Channelling crystal

Accumulation crystal   Tabular crystal   Transmitter crystal

Rock Crystal is also excellent for combining in an application with other crystals, as it amplifies their strength.

Rose Quartz

Rose Quartz is another well-known crystal, and is often used for countering interference. Usually, no distinction is made between technical radiation and geopathic stress radiation from the earth with regards to the use of Rose Quartz. This means it is applied both for electromagnetic stress as well as for stress from an earth source, such as water veins and similar. It is often recommended to place an unworked Rose Quartz crystal beside or under the bed, or on the electrical apparatus in question, in order to 'earth' the radiation.

However, the term 'earthing' in this circumstance is a little misleading. It is possible to earth electrical and electro-magnetic fields as a shielding measure, but from a physical perspective a crystal can never accomplish this. Even from an energetic standpoint the justification for this argument is tenuous at best.

Aside from that, Rose Quartz is a wonderful crystal. When analysed with a dowsing rod or a pendulum, you can see that it emits almost exclusively positive oscillations. In principle this means that it influences the climate of a room in a positive manner and thus, energetically, can create a certain balance for disturbances that otherwise cannot be removed. It can therefore make the interfering radiation more bearable for us for a certain time, by having a harmonising effect mentally and spiritually.

But the problem is (as with all other crystals) that its influence is restricted and become exhausted at some point. Depending on the strength and the type of radiation, it will only work for hours or days, then the effect turns into its opposite. This means that in order to utilise a crystal's potential purposefully and sensibly, you need to check its effect at least daily and then regularly cleanse and recharge the crystal. Here too, the following applies: the less radiation is actually present, the longer the crystal will retain its positive effect!

The truth is that effective energetic suppression is usually at least as time-consuming as changing your sleeping location or employing physical building biology measures to reduce radiation. In addition, the positive energetic effect of Rose Quartz can only unfold properly over longer periods if the physical causes of the radiation have been reduced as much as possible. Rose Quartz should therefore only be used in combination with building biology measures for reducing radiation. Then its harmonising effect will unfold optimally.

Rose Quartz also radiates a quality that makes you feel awake. So, if you have trouble getting to sleep or sleeping through the night, don't lay Rose Quartz near your bed!

Rose Quartz also improves sensitivity; heightens empathic responses, the ability to love and to be helpful; harmonises the heart rhythm and strengthens the heart.

Black Tourmaline (Schorl)
Tourmaline Quartz (Schorl in Quartz)

Black Tourmaline is considered to be the classic crystal of protection, and essentially protects from outside influences.

This applies mainly to energetic influences.

It is often recommended to lay this Quartz between yourself and the source of radiation, for example the monitor screen. But, as with all other crystals, it does not physically shield you, so we recommend wearing it on the body where its positive energetic effect may unfold more successfully. If you have exhausted all the building biology measures, Black Tourmaline may help to make the remaining radiation more bearable by dissolving blockages in the flow of energy.

For example, Tourmaline can be extremely effective if you are travelling and have to be in rooms that are subjected to high levels of radiation. A necklace of Black Tourmaline, for example, may help to compensate for the effects of radiation, for a limited amount of time.

All types of Tourmaline have an essentially stimulating effect on the energy flow of the body, with Black Tourmaline being the most important one. It also improves connection and communication throughout the various levels of function in the human organism, connecting spirit, soul, mind and body into a harmonious whole – and what better prerequisite could there be for a healthy life.

One of the main problems with electromagnetic stress is that the resulting radiation substantially affects the communications processes within the body. For the complex system of the human body to function, the activities of the cells, the organs and the organ systems need to be able to exchange information on a continuous basis in order to coordinate those activities. In this context, radiation is a significant disturbing impulse, and optimal exchange of information is prevented. This, in turn, causes control disruptions, energetic blockages and finally illness.

Black Tourmaline helps to re-establish the energy flow and the healthy exchange of information, and even acts as a preventative for larger energy flow disruptions.

Its black colour is, in itself, indicative of setting a boundary. Its other characteristics, too, suit the symptoms caused by electromagnetic stress.

Tourmaline alleviates stress, helps with muscle tension and pain, and encourages sleep.

Within **Tourmaline Quartz**, fine Tourmaline needles are captured in Rock crystal. In principle, it works in the same way as Black Tourmaline.

It dissolves stress, tension and hardening. It has an enlivening, activating effect – more so even than Black Tourmaline – and therefore helps you find equilibrium between tension and relaxation. In this state the body is able to react optimally and appropriately to external influences, and to balance disturbances.

Smoky Quartz/Morion

Smoky Quartz is formed under the influence of radioactive radiation, which is emitted from the surrounding rock. It helps make you resistant to radiation and alleviates radiation damage. It has a very strong relaxing effect, and is considered to be the classic crystal against stress.

Electromagnetic pollution in particular causes a constant stress reaction in the body, a kind of permanent state of alarm that continues until all energy reserves are exhausted. The first symptoms are often restlessness, irritability, nervousness, sleep disturbances, tension, headaches, and digestive problems. Usually, the result is a chronic feeling of exhaustion and lowered immune response, which then opens the door to further disease.

In such cases, Smoky Quartz may help to dissolve the tension. It heightens your ability to withstand stress and strengthens the nerves, and you become less sensitive to all external influences.

Smoky Quartz is excellent for acute symptoms of radiation stress. In the long term, though, it cannot compensate for severe stress. The causes of stress need to be addressed, that is, the radiation stress needs to be reduced to a level where the body can manage without the crystal.

The **Morion** is a special, dark (almost black) Smoky Quartz, which has been exposed to particularly strong radiation and is therefore extremely good for use in cases of radiation influence.

Smoky Quartz should be worn directly on the body for prolonged periods. It can also be placed on painful or tense points on the body. For relaxation use two larger tumbled crystals, or hold a crystal in each hand.

Tektite

Tektite is formed when a large meteorite hits the Earth. Both the meteorite and the earthly rock suddenly evaporate. The explosion causes molten rock splashes to be flung out, which then solidify in the air.

Tektite encourages the realisation that you are a spiritual being, and strengthens your empathetic and clairvoyant abilities. It imparts spontaneity, impulsiveness and new ideas, and it liberates you from anxiety and attachment to material things.

Tektite appears to have a very positive influence on stress caused by electromagnetic pollution, especially that which is caused by high frequency radiation (mobile phones, cordless telephones, etc.). Kinesiological tests show that the body appears to react less strongly to a mobile phone conversation when one is carrying Tektite. It would seem, then, that Tektite can improve your ability to cope with radiation, at least for a short time. It helps compensate for the radiation; however, that does not mean the radiation is harmless or does not leach energy from the body. Even with a Tektite, in the long run frequent exposure to radiation stress will lead to exhaustion of the body's energy reserves. Tektite can be used to cope with unavoidable stress in occasional circumstances, but don't be tempted to expose yourself unnecessarily to damaging radiation!

Generally, Tektite is indicated to help with all strong physical, mental and spiritual stress, in order to 'switch off', so to speak. So, in cases of severe stress you can also use it to create some 'space' for a while, thus giving yourself time to act.

This will not work for the long term, however. You will still need to identify and remove the causes of the stress.

On a physical level, Tektite crystals encourage healing processes, and they do so by bringing the causes of the illness into consciousness. They are especially helpful with infectious diseases.

Tip: When the Crystal Healing Association tested Tektite, it found that the crystal may actually activate latent or potential diseases. In the end this may be viewed as part of the healing process, but may also be rather unpleasant if you aren't expecting it!

Difficulties with getting to sleep and periods of disturbed sleep may be alleviated and even healed with Tektite. Try drinking Tektite water before going to sleep, and laying a Tektite crystal under your pillow.

Immune System

Another important subject in connection with electromagnetic pollution is its effects on the body's immune system. It has been proven that electromagnetic pollution weakens the immune defences and actually opens the door to infections and severe illnesses.

The function of the immune system is extremely complex, and various aspects play a part on the different levels of being – physical, mental and spiritual. That is why you will not find a separate chapter on the subject; the issues and remedies addressed in the following chapters as a whole provide the foundation for a healthy and properly functioning immune system.

Many crystals are capable of fortifying the immune system. As a rule, they do so by aiding one of the aspects described in the following chapters.

Protection and Boundary Setting

The ability to create proper boundaries plays an essential role in maintaining good health and ensuring the wellbeing of a living organism. The better you are able to set boundaries, the better you are protected from outside influences. This is most easily perceived on a physical level. The skin and the mucous membranes are responsible for preventing foreign substances from entering the body. If the skin is damaged, or the mucous membranes can no longer properly fulfil their functions, disease-causing organisms can invade the body and damage it. But protecting yourself from external influences on the mental and spiritual levels is equally essential to remaining healthy. The different levels are closely connected. Experience shows that humans who have a well developed ability to delimit themselves emotionally and spiritually usually have a good immune system, and are not quickly shaken out of a state of equilibrium by external influences. Thus, as a rule, they also react less sensitively to electromagnetic pollution.

In the following you will find descriptions of several crystals that are able to encourage positive boundary setting abilities on the physical, mental and spiritual levels. Most of them also fortify the immune system.

Agate (→ Immune System, Stability)
The world of Agates is an extensive one, and, depending on their signature or marking, each will have an affect on specific areas of the body. Regularly-banded Agates are particularly suitable as protection from electromagnetic pollution. They balance the aura and the energetic bodies, and ensure that a strong, protective, enveloping shield is created on the energetic plane.

   Agate encourages spiritualisation, focus, concentration, and the art of consciously dealing with life experiences. In this way Agate allows you to grow and mature spiritually, and leads to inner stability and a proper sense of reality. It dissolves internal tension and lends protection, security and safety, thus rendering you more stable in the face of external influences. Generally it imparts a logical, pragmatic and well-grounded attitude to life.

Thunder eggs, *also called Star Agates or amulet stones,* stimulate the liver (detoxification) and the immune system. They stabilise the physical and mental constitution.

Mica (→ Detoxification)

All minerals in the Mica group provide good protective crystals, as do other rock types containing large proportions of Mica. They help with boundary setting, and support a sense of your own identity and autonomy. They also have a detoxifying effect.

The following mica-containing crystals are particularly interesting in connection with the symptoms of electromagnetic stress:

Biotite (→ Metabolism, Detoxification)

Biotite lenses are considered to be the traditional protective crystals in Portugal, which is where they are found. Biotite fortifies your will for the task of self-realisation; it helps to liberate you from being determined by others, and also from the demands of others. It motivates you to realise your own ideas, and to make decisions. On the physical level it works as a detoxifying crystal, as do all crystals containing Mica; it balances over-acidification and works well for rheumatism, gout and sciatica.

Lepidolite (Mica containing Lithium)
(→ Metabolism, Detoxification)

Lepidolite protects from external influences and helps with boundary setting. It encourages autonomy and self-discipline. For painful conditions, which may arise in connection with electromagnetic stress, Lepidolite can be applied to alleviate neuralgic pain, for example with sciatica and joint problems.

It also has a detoxifying effect, balances over-acidification, and stimulates the cleansing processes of the skin and connective tissues.

Fuchsite (→ Immune System, Detoxification)

Fuchsite is a Mica that contains Chromium. It helps with boundary setting, but also with remaining alert and attentive to the external world. It is possible to view worries from a certain distance, without denying them. Fuchsite encourages creative problem-solving, and keeps the spirit and body flexible. Especially important in terms of electromagnetic stress, Fuchsite fortifies the immune system and encourages detoxification. It alleviates sudden-onset inflammations, and helps with allergies and other conditions that produce skin eruptions with itching and scaliness.

Fuchsite with Ruby is particularly interesting in connection with electromagnetic pollution as the protective and detoxifying effects of the Fuchsite merge with the vitalising and fortifying powers of Ruby (see also Ruby, page 36).

Aventurine (→ Harmonisation and Balance, Immune System, Detoxification)

Aventurine is a type of crystal that contains both Quartz and Fuchsite, and so it belongs among the crystals containing Mica. It is described in detail in the *Harmonisation and Balance* chapter.

Heliotrope (→ Immune System, Strength, Metabolism, Detoxification)

Heliotrope is a green Chalcedony with inclusions of yellow and red Jasper. It helps you to protect yourself, set boundaries, and keep at bay unwanted external influences. It lends flexibility and the ability to adapt without compromising your own point of view. In cases of exhaustion and tiredness it lends strength, while at the same time relieving irritability and nervousness. On a physical level, Heliotrope is also one of the best immune-fortifying crystals, especially in cases of acute infection. It stimulates the lymph flow and metabolism, and detoxifies and neutralises over-acidification.

Serpentine (→ Harmonisation and Balance,
  Metabolism)

Serpentine is another classic protective crystal. Due to its layered structure, it strengthens the ability to set boundaries. Physically it has a cramp-relieving effect and works against over-acidification. It also helps balance mood swings and imparts inner peace.

Turquoise (→ Harmonisation and Balance,
  Metabolism, Detoxification)
Turquoise is one of the best known protective crystals. It makes you less sensitive to external influences by strengthening your own identity and mobilising energy reserves. It makes you conscious of being 'at the root' of your life and fate, and helps you to find the strength and the courage to bring about changes if they become necessary. So, it helps you to take your life into your own hands and control it from a place of personal power. Turquoise also balances mood swings. Especially helpful in terms of electromagnetic stress, Turquoise has a pain-relieving effect, dissolves cramps, soothes inflammations, detoxifies, and dissolves acidification.

Additional crystals for protection and boundary setting:

Jade (Jadeite/Nephrite) (→ **Harmonisation and Balance,**
  Metabolism, Elimination)

Strengthening Life Energy – Power and Vitality

Stressing the body with electromagnetic pollution will drain strength from the body and, in the end, also from the soul. The following crystals may help mobilise your energy reserves for a while, without at the same time stimulating too strongly or amplifying the stress. They impart vitality and the energy to deal with stressful situations more easily.

The application of these crystals makes sense even in situations where electromagnetic stress has been present for a long time, and where long-term stress has led to serious illness or extensive physical and mental exhaustion.

Garnet (→ Immune System, Regeneration, Metabolism)
Garnet has a general regenerative quality and strengthens resistance. It fortifies the will and, in times of crisis, lends stamina and endurance, courage and trust. It helps you glimpse the light at the end of the tunnel, and, when it seems that nothing is working, it helps you overcome your doubts and do what is necessary.

When severe stress from electromagnetic pollution has been present for some time, many people reach a point where they can no longer carry on, especially if the stress has not been recognised, and doctors can find no cause for the often severe symptoms.

Many patients for whom all treatment options have failed find themselves put into the 'psycho-corner', and subsequently lose all hope of improvement or cure. In such cases, Garnet may lend renewed hope and confidence. It may help the patient find their own path to recovery and overcome external resistance.

Above all, Garnet fortifies the body's powers of regeneration and removes energetic blockages. It stimulates the metabolism and improves the consistency of each of the body's fluids. It stabilises the blood circulation, fortifies the immune system, and accelerates the healing of internal and external injuries (wounds).

Ruby (→ Immune System, Metabolism)

Ruby imparts strength and 'joie de vivre', vitality and dynamism, but without over-stimulating you into hyper-activity. It improves productivity, efficiency and self-confidence. It helps in cases of discouragement and exhaustion, which may also have arisen as consequences of long-term stress, for example from electro-magnetic pollution. Ruby may also awaken new initiatives and a readi-ness to take action in those who have tried many things to heal their suffering and have subsequently lost hope.

Physically, Ruby stimulates the spleen, the adrenals and the circula-tion. It supports the immune system and helps with combating infectious diseases. It activates the entire metabolism and may help with recover-ing the organism's ability to react, so that other natural measures will once again prove effective.

Red Jasper

Red Jasper brings dynamism and activity, but without the impulsiveness sometimes associated with Ruby.

It stimulates the circulation and the body's energy flow. Jasper encourages will power, courage and a readiness for conflict, therefore making it easier to initiate necessary changes and to persevere with a therapy already underway.

Hematite

Hematite lends strength, vitality and liveliness. It is effec-tive almost exclusively on the physical level. It improves the gut's ability to absorb iron and supports the formation of red blood corpuscles, thereby improving the overall supply of oxygen to the entire body.

Tiger Iron

Tiger Iron consists of alternating layers (bands) of Tiger Eye, Jasper and Hematite, and combines the positive qualities of all three crystals. It heightens vitality, and lends strength, dynamism and endurance. It therefore helps with lack of iron (anaemia), tiredness and exhaustion. It encourages the absorption of iron and the formation of red blood corpuscles, and also the supply of oxygen to the body. Tiger Iron has a very rapid effect and can therefore be applied for acute states of low energy.

Mookaite (→ Immune system, Stability)

Mookaite is a coloured Chert, which is a mixture of Opal and Jasper. In Australia it is still employed by the original inhabitants as an energising healing stone.

It imparts vitality and dynamism together with internal focus, peace and equilibrium. It also lends liveliness, which is realised in harmonious activity, but without draining the body's resources. Mookaite helps you discern what would be the right amount of input in a given situation, and encourages you to only do as much as is needed and is good for you. That way, ideas and projects can be realised with fun and joy.

Physically, Mookaite's foremost effect is cleansing the blood in the liver and spleen. It fortifies the body's vitality and the immune system. It also helps stabilise health in the long term. Like Jasper, Mookaite also heightens vitality and the strength of the whole body. It should be worn for an extended period of time in order to unfold its full effect.

Strengthening the Centre – Stability

Stressful situations are best handled when you are fully aware of your own resources and can face the situation with internal calm and focus. The crystals described in the following section strengthen your 'centre' and earth-connectedness. They encourage a relaxed attitude, stability and endurance, and thus provide the optimal basis for dealing with environmental stresses.

Dendritic Agate (Tree Agate) (→ Immune System)
Dendritic Agate imparts persistence, security, stability and endurance, even in unpleasant situations, and makes you aware of your own strength. Thus it helps with taking on challenges and dealing with them. It encourages vitality in the body and stable good health. Dendritic Agate fortifies resistance and the immune system and helps with susceptibility to infection. It should be worn for an extended period of time in order to fully unfold its effect.

Brown and yellow Jasper (→ Immune System)
Brown and yellow Jasper mainly support endurance and stamina. They encourage focus and impart inner calm, while fortifying the immune system long-term. They are especially helpful with diseases of the gut and the digestive organs.

Fossil Wood (→ Metabolism)
Fossil Wood encourages a proper sense of reality and has a grounding effect.

It imparts centring and calm focus, then releases energy over the long term without exhausting the body's reserves. It helps you become aware of your body's signals – to listen and respond to them – and it lends a sense of wellbeing and an enjoyment of the simple things in life. Physically, Fossil Wood stabilises good health and imparts energy, as well as aiding recovery. It activates the metabolism and calms the nerves, and is therefore very beneficial in cases of feeling 'wound up', restless, and nervous – symptoms that often arise in a body burdened by electro-magnetic stress.

Opalised Fossil Wood also encourages detoxification and elimination.

Additional crystals for stability:

Agate (→ Protection and Boundary Setting, Immune System)

Star Agate (→ Protection and Boundary Setting, Immune System, Detoxification)

Mookaite (→ Strength and Vitality, Immune System)

Ocean Jasper (→ Regeneration, Immune System, Detoxification)

Regeneration

Burdening caused by stress from electromagnetic pollution can lead a person to the limits of his or her physical and mental ability to with-stand stress, and may, in the long term, even trigger serious illnesses. Especially if health is affected for a long time and the causes are recog-nised late or not at all, exhaustion and resignation will often gain the upper hand. Thankfully, there are some crystals that can help with regaining courage, and help stimulate the organism's powers of regen-eration on both the physical and mental levels.

Ocean Jasper (→ Immune System, Stability, Detoxification)

Strictly-speaking, Ocean Jasper is not a Jasper at all, but rather a Rhyolite containing Quartz, which means it is a volcanic crystal. Sometimes it is also referred to as Ocean Agate.

It encourages a positive outlook on life and helps you to withstand stress and remain calm through self-acceptance. Ocean Jasper also encourages healthy sleep. Physically, it strengthens the immune system and promotes detoxification, and helps with flu, stubborn colds, cysts and tumours. Subsequently, it is also a valuable helper for alleviating the consequences of electromagnetic stress.

Epidote (→ Immune System)

Epidote helps you recognise your own condition and makes you conscious of actual reality. It encourages measured processes of change, and the patience required for a realistic translation of your own wishes and goals into reality. It also encourages recuperation and regeneration on all levels – physical, mental and spiritual. It fortifies the capacity for being productive and efficient, strengthens the constitution, has a general building-up and fortifying effect, and supports all healing processes. Thus Epidote is able to stabilise the immune system and stimulate the liver function and the digestive processes.

Epidote can also be successfully applied as a regenerating mineral after severe colds or serious stress. It will also lend the patience needed to allow the recuperation and building-up processes to take place, enabling a realistic evaluation of what is possible and what would be too demanding and therefore bring about a relapse.

Zoisite (→ Immune System, Metabolism, Detoxification)

Zoisite helps in overcoming resignation and destructive mental attitudes. It encourages creativity and an ability to take your life into your own hands. It encourages the development of your wishes and ideas, and helps liberate you from a tendency to over-adapt to others or to be determined by external factors.

Physically, it stimulates the forces of regeneration in the cells and of the entire organism, and also encourages recuperation after great stress and serious illnesses. It also helps with detoxification and with neutralising over-acidification. Zoisite inhibits inflammations and strengthens the immune system.

Zoisite is also available in the trade as **Ruby with Zoisite**. Both crystals complement the other's effects very well, especially when they are applied for problems due to electromagnetic pollution.

Zoisite unfolds its effects slowly and should therefore be worn for longer periods with direct skin contact.

Additional crystals for regeneration:
Garnet (→ Strength, Immune System, Metabolism)
Brown Tourmaline (Dravite) (→ Harmonisation and Balance, Metabolism, Autonomic Nervous System)
Emerald (→ Detoxification, Metabolism, Immune System, Harmonisation and Balance)

Harmonisation and Balance

Electromagnetic stress is a strong interference impulse that causes imbalance in both the body and the psyche. The natural regulatory systems in the body go haywire and, in the long term, this also has an effect on emotional balance. Electromagnetic stress favours extremes – for example, over-reaction of the immune system in the form of allergies and auto-immune illnesses or a weakened immune system; hormonal over- or under-production, often also connected with severe mood swings; and a multitude of other issues. In such cases, the crystals listed below may have a balancing effect and help harmonise physical and mental over-reactions.

Jade (Jadeite/Nephrite) (→ Protection and Boundary Setting, Metabolism, Elimination)
The general term 'Jade' actually covers two very different minerals, Jadeite and Nephrite, which have very similar effects. Jadeite

is extremely rare, and most crystals referred to as Jade are actually Nephrite.

Jade contains different mineral substances, some stimulating, some calming. Thus Jade imparts the balance necessary in life, activating in times of lethargy and calming in times of stress or irritability. In the long term it brings a stable condition of inner balance, and a sense of measure in all things. At the same time, Jade also makes you mentally active and proactive. It helps strengthen your own sense of identity, and is also considered a traditional protective crystal against external attack.

Physically, Jade stimulates kidney function and thus balances the levels of water, salts, and acid/alkaline fluids. It stimulates the nervous system and regulates the function of the adrenals. It therefore has a balancing effect on the production of the stress hormones adrenaline and noradrenaline, which place the body in a state of readiness in an emergency (the fight or flight response). An increased release of these hormones often plays an important role in the reaction to electromagnetic pollution. In such cases, Jade is able to provide balance and restore the organism's ability to react, so that the body is better able to deal with illness and therapy blockages.

Tourmaline (→ Metabolism, Autonomic
   Nervous System)

Tourmaline is one of the most diverse crystals of the mineral kingdom as it occurs in many different colours. Thus, according to its colour, Tourmaline possesses a wide spectrum of healing effects. In connection with balance and harmony it is the multi-coloured Tourmaline that is of particular interest. It helps bring the spirit, psyche, intellect and body into a harmonious whole. It makes you permeable and flexible, stimulates the

energy flow in the meridians, and helps dissolve blockages. Physically, it has a building-up effect and is stimulating in cases of weakness. It harmonises the nerves, the metabolism, the hormonal glands, and the immune system.

In the case of multi-coloured Tourmalines, combinations of the following colours are particularly recommended:

Rubellite (red Tourmaline) improves the energy flow and the conductivity of the nerves. It strengthens the functions of the sexual organs, and encourages a good blood supply and blood cleansing in the spleen and the liver. **Verdelite (green Tourmaline)** also fortifies the heart and has a detoxifying effect. It also supports elimination. **Dravite (brown-yellow Tourmaline)** stimulates the regenerative powers of the cells, the tissues and the organs.

Amazonite (→ Autonomic Nervous System, Metabolism)
Physically, Amazonite regulates metabolic problems and has a relaxing and cramp-dissolving effect. It strengthens the nerves and harmonises the autonomic nervous system and the internal organs. Mentally and spiritually, Amazonite balances mood swings. It has a calming effect and imparts trust. In addition, Amazonite supports self-determination and helps you rid yourself of the feeling that you are a victim of a cruel fate. Thus it stimulates you to take control of your own life.

Aventurine (→ Immune System, Detoxification, Protection and Boundary Setting)
Aventurine is a Quartz that obtains its green, glittering appearance through inclusions of Fuchsite. It optimally combines the effects of Quartz (see Rock Crystal) and Fuchsite.

Time and again Aventurine has proven effective for the prevention and healing of radiation damage. It imparts resistance to radiation stress and quickly alleviates unpleasant side effects such as headaches and other pain, nervous complaints, autonomic nervous problems and skin irritations.

It helps with nervousness, stress and sleep disorders, and relaxes the body and the psyche. It also liberates you from external influences and demands. Aventurine is therefore an outstanding crystal in cases of electromagnetic pollution burdening, which places the body and psyche under constant stress and may often lead to the aforementioned symptoms. Aventurine is particularly helpful if you are the type of person who places great demands upon yourself and tends to expect too much of yourself. It also helps you 'switch off' if you are worrying too much about a potential stress and its consequences.

Additional crystals for harmonisation and balance:

Serpentine (→ Protection and Boundary Setting, Metabolism)

Emerald (→ Detoxification, Metabolism, Immune System, Regeneration)

Rose Quartz (→ the classic electromagnetic pollution crystal)

Sunstone (→ Fortification of the Autonomic Nervous System)

Amber (→ Fortification of the Autonomic Nervous System)

Strengthening the Autonomic Nervous System

Ametrine (→ Metabolism, Autonomic Nervous System)
Ametrine is a combination of Amethyst and Citrine in a single mineral. It lends creativity, optimism, and 'joie de vivre', and a sense of control over your own life. On the mental level it encourages harmony and emotional wellbeing, which will also prevail in stressful situations. Physically, it has a cleansing effect and activates the cellular metabolism, which is often severely disrupted through burdening from electromagnetic stress. Ametrine also strengthens the autonomic nervous system and harmonises the interplay between the internal organs. Thus it harmonises and vitalises the entire organism.

Sunstone (→ Harmonisation)
Sunstone activates your own healing powers. It stimulates
the autonomic nervous system and ensures a harmonious
interplay among the organs. Mentally and spiritually Sunstone lends
'joie de vivre' and optimism. It lightens the mood and is anti-depressive,
and increases one's sense of self-worth and self confidence.

Amber (→ Harmonisation)
Amber imparts a carefree disposition, happiness and trust.
It lends a sunny disposition and increases your belief in
yourself. You are then better able to rest in your centre,
and react flexibly to external conditions without losing your centre.
Physically, Amber helps with joint problems and fortifies the mucous
membranes. It stimulates wound healing, helps with stomach, spleen
and kidney complaints, and has a positive effect on the liver and the
gall bladder.

Additional crystals for fortifying the autonomic nervous system
Amazonite (→ Harmonisation and Balance, Metabolism)
Tourmaline (→ Harmonisation and Balance, Metabolism)

The Metabolism and Detoxification

The term 'metabolism' covers the absorption, transportation and
chemical transformation of substances in an organism, and the elimination of metabolic waste products to the environment. This includes,
for example, respiration, digestion, and many other bodily processes in
which one substance is transformed into another. These events are
very complex and may well become disturbed through electromagnetic
pollution burdening. Such a disturbance causes an increased produc-

tion of waste products from incomplete or compromised transformation processes, such as free radicals and damaging acids. These waste products are transported not only by the blood, but also by 'white blood', or lymph fluids.

The waste products are present in the spaces between the cells, in what is called the 'connective tissues', and are transported via the lymph channels to the organs of elimination. Metabolic waste products are also stored temporarily between the connective tissues; however, if too many waste products are stored they 'clog up' the connective tissues, and the lymph fluids no longer eliminate them. The tissues become clogged with toxic waste and the entire organism becomes over-acidic. A well-functioning metabolism and well-functioning lymph flow are indispensable prerequisites for maintaining good health.

As already mentioned above, electromagnetic stress may interfere considerably with metabolic processes and also impair the lymphatic flow.

Electromagnetic pollution causes over-acidification of the tissues and can therefore bring with it some well-known consequences: pain, tension, tiredness, chronic inflammations, immune weakness, hair loss, osteoporosis, the encouragement of cancerous conditions, and more.

The following provides descriptions of crystals that may be helpful for these problems:

The Chalcedony Family

Generally, Chalcedony crystals impart lightness, openness, the ability to make friends easily, and improved communication.

Blue Chalcedony, the best known representative of the Chalcedony family, encourages flexibility, helps with inner resistance, and imparts inner calm.

Physically, blue Chalcedony and banded Chalcedony stimulate the flow of bodily fluids, especially the lymph flow, and thereby help reduce water retention in the tissues (oedemas), eliminate metabolic waste products, and strengthen the immune system. If the heart function also needs strengthening, **pink Chalcedony** may also be used. For low blood pressure, **red Chalcedony** has a stimulating effect on the circulation.

Copper Chalcedony also stimulates the copper metabolism and the detoxification processes of the liver.

Dendritic Agate (→ Detoxification)

Dendritic Agate has a detoxifying effect and encourages the elimination of waste products, which are incompletely processed metabolic products from the tissues.

Opalite (→ Detoxification)

Opalite encourages sociability and good contact with your surroundings and other people. Physically it fortifies the mucous membranes.

It stimulates the function of the lungs, encourages the absorption of oxygen, and helps with tenacious common cold symptoms and damage from smoking. It encourages waste elimination, detoxification processes and digestive elimination, while also cleansing the connective tissues, intestines and mucous membranes.

Additional crystals for the metabolism and elimination processes

Turquoise (→ **Protection and Boundary Setting**, Detoxification)

Heliotrope (→ **Protection and Boundary Setting**, Immune System, Energy, Detoxification)

Serpentine (→ **Protection and Boundary Setting**, Harmonisation and Balance)

Garnet (→ **Regeneration**, Immune System)

Zoisite (→ **Regeneration**, Immune System, Detoxification)

Ruby in Zoisite (→ **Regeneration**, Immune System, Detoxification, Power and Vitality)

Ametrine (→ **Autonomic Nervous System**, Harmonisation, Detoxification)

coloured Tourmaline (→ **Balance and Harmonisation**, Immune System, Autonomic Nervous System)

Amazonite (→ **Balance and Harmonisation**, Autonomic Nervous System)

Detoxification and Elimination

An increased sensitivity to electromagnetic pollution can come about through multiple stresses on the body resulting from exposure to other toxic substances; for example, exposure to heavy metals from the environment or from amalgam tooth fillings. Detoxification of the body generally results in a noticeable decrease in stress symptoms, and the crystals described here can help set the process in motion. We have chosen the crystals that tend to have a gentle effect and are physically and mentally stabilising, and will usually not bring about violent detoxification reactions. That said, take care if you are already suffering from serious illness, or if you know you have been severely exposed to toxins. Existing symptoms may drastically worsen during a detoxification of the organism, or even cause symptoms of previous illnesses to return. In such cases, you should consult a physician or natural medicine practitioner if you wish to apply these crystals.

Chrysoprase (→ Metabolism and Elimination)

Chrysoprase belongs to the Chalcedony family. It therefore improves the flow properties of bodily fluids, especially those of the lymph, and encourages elimination of waste products.

Through its inclusion of nickel, which also lends it that apple-green colouring, Chrysoprase has a strong detoxifying effect. Even the elimination of heavy metals and other substances that do not dissolve easily is stimulated by this crystal. It is also excellent for supporting the liver. Chrysoprase helps with illnesses that arise as a consequence of poisoning, and is also helpful with allergies, skin diseases and rheumatism.

On mental and spiritual levels, Chrysoprase has a cleansing and dissolving effect. It helps you work through stressful experiences and to overcome negative feelings, to liberate you from unhelpful thoughts, and to direct your attention to positive events. It imparts feelings of trust and security. It also helps you 'sort yourself out', so to speak, and to experience an all-encompassing feeling of coherence and deep trust that comes from being part of a greater whole, a whole to which you can contribute in ways that are in keeping with your self and your capabilities.

Green Garnet (→ Metabolism, Regeneration)

The green varieties of Garnet, Tsavorite and Uvarovite, are particularly stimulating for detoxification, and also have an anti-inflammatory effect. Tsavorite, in particular, also brings new strength in life's difficult times and helps you face problems and overcome difficulties.

For mental-spiritual effects, see also the section on Garnet under *Strengthing Life Energy*.

Emerald (→ Metabolism, Immune System, Regeneration, Harmonisation)

Emerald lends alertness, clarity, far-sightedness, and encourages a sense of beauty, aesthetics, harmony and justice. It imparts a new orientation in life-crisis situations and supports you in identifying goals and finding meaning.

Emerald accelerates spiritual growth and strengthens the ability to regenerate and rejuvenate. Emerald works particularly well with inflammations of the upper respiratory tract and nasal sinus cavities. It stimulates liver function, encourages detoxification and de-acidification, and helps with typical acid-based problems such as rheumatism or gout. It alleviates pain and strengthens the immune system.

Additional crystals for detoxification and elimination:

Turquoise (→ Protection and Boundary Setting, Metabolism)

(Mica → Protection and Boundary Setting)

Lepidolite (→ Protection and Boundary Setting, Metabolism and Detoxification)

Fuchsite (→ Protection and Boundary Setting, Metabolism and Detoxification)

Aventurine (→ Protection and Boundary Setting, Immune System)

Zoisite (→ Regeneration, Metabolism, Immune System)

Ruby in Zoisite (→ Regeneration, Immune System, Metabolism, Power and Vitality)

Ocean Jasper (→ Stability, Immune System, Detoxification, Regeneration)

Star Agate (→ Stability Immune System, Protection and Boundary Setting)

Fossil Wood, opalised (→ Stability, Metabolism and Detoxification)

Jade (Jadeite/Nephrite) (→ Harmonisation and Balance, Metabolism)

Green Tourmaline (Verdelite) (→ Harmonisation and Balance, Metabolism, Autonomic Nervous System)

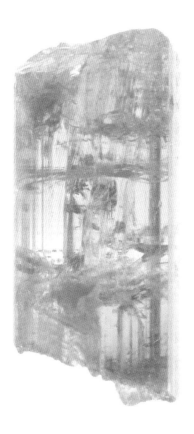

Choosing the Right Crystal

The Analytical Approach

What are the problems you are experiencing? If there are several, which are the most prominent? First, try to narrow down the list of crystals by choosing an overall subject heading; for example, 'Protection and Boundary Setting', 'Power and Stability', 'Regeneration', and so on. Then, within the relevant section, look for the crystal that best fits your symptoms. You will find an index of all symptoms and suitable crystals in the Appendix.

The Intuitive Approach

As we already stated at the beginning, the healing power of crystals rests in their energetic effects. The phenomenon of resonance plays a major role.

Resonance is derived from the Latin 'resonare', which means something like 'vibrating with'. For example, if there are two guitars in the same room and you pluck a string on the first guitar, the same string on the second guitar will begin to resonate and even produce a sound, providing both strings are tuned to the same note. This means that one string stimulates the other to vibrate along with it, and thus be in a state of resonance.

The same applies to living organisms, and also in the field of energetic healing. For example, if the vibration of a healing substance corresponds exactly with an illness or a symptom, then a great effect can be achieved, even with vibrations so subtle they are no longer physically measurable. The workings of homeopathy and of the Bach flower remedies are based on this principle. The greatest effect and the deepest levels of healing are achieved when the vibrations of the healing substance correspond with the mood, the character, and the momentary spiritual/mental condition of the patient.

It is then that the strongest possible resonance is achieved – physically, mentally and spiritually.

You can make use of this resonance principle to find the right crystals (or several crystals) for your own use. Everyone can sense resonance. It is that feeling of being addressed by or attracted to something spontaneously and without thinking about it. For example, you might think, 'Oh, yes, that's it', or simply find something attractive or interesting. Perhaps you stop at a particular sentence, or at the sight of something, and only then begin to think about it. Or maybe you simply feel it physically, as a sensation in your physical centre or in the area of your heart.

Simply follow that feeling or that spontaneous moment of interest. Perhaps in the course of reading this little book you may have experienced such moments. Try and remember which crystals or keywords caught your interest.

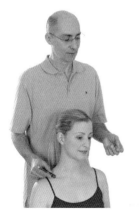

Testing with a single dowsing rod

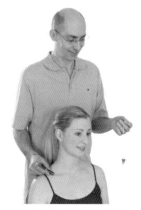

Testing with a pendulum

If you can't remember specifically, peruse all the overall subject headings again and choose one or two of them. Then read a few of the descriptions of crystals and pay attention to which crystal spontaneously appeals to you.

With the help of a pendulum or a single dowsing rod it is possible to make that resonance visible. This is especially meaningful if you have not yet had the experience of paying attention to your own intuition and the subtle signals from your body and soul. Working with a pendulum or a dowsing rod is a great way to access your own intuition when choosing the right crystal.

The best results come about by using a combination of the analytical and intuitive approaches. If both results converge, then you will have found the best crystal to use.

Sometimes this will be quite easy and you will immediately know which crystal is needed, but other times it may be difficult to set priorities and many different crystals will appear to fit the situation. Then it may make sense to enlist the help of a professional crystal consultant.

The Application of Crystals

There are many ways to apply the power of crystals. For the purposes outlined in this book, we recommend wearing the relevant crystal for a while with skin contact. For example, it can be stuck on in the form of a tumbled crystal, or a raw crystal, or worn as a pendant or a necklace. The duration of application will vary in individual cases and will also depend on the type of crystal being used. Some crystals unfold their effects relatively quickly, while others have to be worn longer in order to feel an effect.

Generally speaking, the crystal should be worn long enough for the symptoms to have disappeared, or for as long as you feel comfortable with it. Sometimes it happens that the crystal disappears, is lost, or you simply no longer think about using it. This probably indicates that the crystal has now done its job.

Cleansing

Crystals that are worn for long periods of time should be regularly cleansed both physically and energetically. For a physical cleansing they can be held in flowing water for a while. For energetic cleansing, you can place your crystal upon or within a piece of Amethyst or Smoky Crystal druse, which has the additional advantage of recharging it energetically. Another possibility is cleansing the crystal with salt. The crystal is laid in a shallow dish with dry salt crystals for 3–4 hours (no longer!). Most crystals cope well with this, but occasionally the procedure may lead to dulling of the surface of polished, shiny crystals. If you want to be absolutely certain no harm will come to your crystals, lay them in a smaller dish and place that dish in a larger one containing salt. This means the crystals have no immediate contact with the salt, but are nevertheless cleansed. More detailed information on cleansing and recharging crystals can be found in the little volume *Purifying Crystals* by Michael Gienger, which is available from Earthdancer Books.

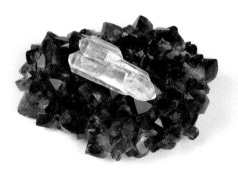

Anti-interference Devices with Crystals

There are a multitude of helpful devices available that utilise crystals for eliminating interference from geopathic radiation or electromagnetic radiation. They usually contain tumbled crystals or granulates made out of the 'classic' anti-interference crystals, or combinations of them. Among these are mats filled with granulated Tourmaline for laying under the bed, pyramids filled with crystals, raw crystals, pendants and amulets, and many more.

Some of these items have been produced with good intentions, but unfortunately many are imposters that use the cheapest tumbled crystal mixture, stuck together with hot glue, inserted into a plug from the electrical retail market, and sold for a lot of money.

Many of the helpful aids on offer are elaborate and expensive. In my opinion, the price/efficiency ratio does not work at all. It makes much more sense to invest in a building biology investigation instead of spending your money on expensive and often ineffective anti-interference devices.

As a rule, a raw crystal or tumbled crystal will be sufficient to achieve the desired effect on the energetic level. If more is needed, a necklace will often work very well. Greater quantity or expense does not necessarily translate into greater effectiveness. As crystals work on an energetic level and are not actually able to decrease radiation or shield you from it, elaborate constructions or the laying of large quantities of crystals under the bed will not provide more elimination of interference than a very ordinary crystal of a good quality.

Adrenals Jade, Ruby

Allergies Aventurine, Chrysoprase

Autonomic nervous system Amazonite, Ametrine, Amber, Charoite, Sunstone, Tourmaline

Blood Garnet, brown and yellow Jasper, Opalite

Boundary setting Agate, Aventurine, Mica, Heliotrope, Jade, Serpentine, Black Tourmaline, Turquoise

Circulation Garnet, Ruby, red Jasper, red Chalcedony, Tiger Iron

Clogged tissues Chalcedony, Chrysoprase, Opalite, opalised Fossil Wood

Cramp Amazonite, Charoite, Serpentine, Turquoise

Detoxification Aventurine, Chrysoprase, Dendritic Agate, Dendritic Chalcedony, Mica, green Garnet, Heliotrope, Jade, Copper Chalcedony, Opalite, Ocean Jasper, Emerald, Star Agate, Turquoise, green Tourmaline, opalised Fossil Wood, Zoisite

Digestion Epidote, brown and yellow Jasper

Drive Ametrine, Charoite, Garnet, Jade, Jasper, Mookaite, Ruby, red Jasper

Energy Rock Crystal, Tiger Iron, Turquoise

Exhaustion Epidote, Heliotrope, Ruby, Tiger Iron, Turquoise

Harmonisation and balance Amazonite, Ametrine, Aventurine, Jade, Mookaite, Rose Quartz, Serpentine, Emerald, Sunstone, Tourmaline

Heart Aventurine, pink Chalcedony, Charoite, Rose Quartz, green Tourmaline

Identity Mica, Turquoise

Immune system Dendritic Agate, Chalcedony, Epidote, Fuchsite, Fuchsite with Ruby, Garnet, Heliotrope, Jasper, Mookaite, Ocean Jasper, Ruby, Emerald, Star Agate, Tourmaline, Zoisite

Inflammation green Garnet, Heliotrope, Emerald, Turquoise, Zoisite

Kidneys Amber, Jade, Serpentine

Liver Epidote, Amber, Chrysoprase, Garnet, Emerald, Star Agate, red Tourmaline

Lungs blue Chalcedony, Opalite

Lymph Heliotrope, Chalcedony, Chrysoprase

Metabolism Amazonite, Ametrine, Chrysoprase, Dendritic Agate, Garnet, Heliotrope, Opalite, Serpentine, Ruby, Tourmaline, Turquoise, Fossil Wood

Over-acidification Charoite, Mica, Heliotrope, Serpentine, Emerald, Turquoise, Zoisite

Mood swings Amazonite, Serpentine, Turquoise

Mucous membranes Amber, Opalite

Nasal sinus cavities Emerald

Nerves Amazonite, Lepidolite, Jade, Smoky Quartz, Tourmaline, Fossil Wood

Nervousness Aventurine, Heliotrope, Serpentine

Pain Rock Crystal, Lepidolite, Smoky Quartz, Turquoise, Tourmaline, Tourmaline Quartz

Power and vitality Epidote, Fuchsite with Ruby, Garnet, Hematite, red Jasper, Mookaite, Ruby, Tiger Iron

Protection Agate, Aventurine, Mica, Heliotrope, Jade, Serpentine, Black Tourmaline, Turquoise

Reality, sense of Agate, Epidote, Fossil Wood

Regeneration Epidote, Garnet, Ocean Jasper, Ruby in Zoisite, Emerald, brown Tourmaline, Zoisite

Relaxation Amazonite, Aventurine, Smoky Quartz

Self confidence Amber, Ruby, Sunstone

Self determination Amazonite, Ametrine, Turquoise, Zoisite

Sleep Aventurine, Ocean Jasper, Tektite

Spleen Amber, Mookaite, Ruby, red Tourmaline

Stability Agate, Star Agate, Dendritic Agate, Amber, Mookaite, Ocean Jasper, Fossil Wood

Stamina Dendritic Agate, Garnet, red, brown and yellow Jasper, Mookaite, Tiger Iron

Stress Aventurine, Charoite, Smoky Quartz, Serpentine, Black Tourmaline

Tiredness Hematite, Heliotrope, Ruby, Tiger Iron

Trust Amazonite, Amber, pink Chalcedony, Chrysoprase, Dendritic Agate, Garnet, Lepidolite

Willpower Garnet, Mookaite, Ruby, red Jasper

Wound healing Amber, Garnet

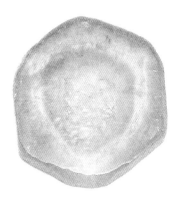

Building Biology contacts and further information

Institute for Bau-Biologie & Ecology
P.O. Box 738
Lyles, TN 37098
United States
1-866-960-0333 (toll-free in US & Canada)
http://buildingbiology.net

Building Biology Environmental Consultant (IBN)
Rainbow Consulting
Katharina Gustavs
5237 Mt. Matheson Rd.
Sooke BC V9Z 1C4 Canada
E-mail: info@buildingbiology.ca
Fax: 250-642-2785
Phone: 250-642-2774
www.buildingbiology.ca

Definition (taken from Wikipedia, the free encyclopaedia):
Building biology (or *Baubiologie* as it was coined in Germany) is a field of
building science that investigates the indoor living environment for a variety
of irritants. Practitioners consider the built environment as something with
which the occupants interact, and believe its functioning can produce a
restful or stressful environment. The major areas focused on by building
biologists are building materials/process, indoor air quality (IAQ) and electromagnetic fields (EMFs).

Thanks

Thank you to Dagmar Fleck and Michael Gienger for their valuable support in the selection and classification of suitable crystals. This little volume could not have come into being without their generosity and willingness to share their expansive knowledge and experience of crystals.

Picture reference

Photos.com/Dragon Design: 8, 11
Barbara Newerla: 9, 25, 26, 28, 31, 32 mid., 34 btm., 35, 36 top, 36 mid., 37, 38 mid., 40 top, 43 top, 43 btm., 45 btm., 49 top, 49 btm., 59
Fotolia.com: 12, 15, 16, 19
Karola Sieber: 22, 29, 33 btm., 34 top, 36 btm., 38 top, 38 btm., 39, 40 btm., 45 top, 47 mid., 47 btm., 50
Dragon Design: 24
Ines Blersch: 32 top, 32 btm., 33 top, 41 top, 42, 44, 47 top, 51, 53, 55

Michael Gienger
Healing Crystals
The A - Z Guide to 430 Gemstones
Paperback, 96 page, ISBN 978-1-84409-067-9

All the important information about 430 healing gemstones in a neat pocket-book!
Michael Gienger, known for his popular introductory work '*Crystal Power, Crystal Heal-ing*', here presents a comprehensive directory of all the gemstones currently in use. In a clear, concise and precise style, with pictures accompanying the text, the author describes the characteristics and healing functions of each crystal.

Michael Gienger
The Healing Crystal First Aid Manual
A practical A to Z of common ailments and illnesses and how they can be best treated with crystal therapy.
288 pages, with 16 colour plates, ISBN 978-1-84409-084-6

This is an easy-to-use A-Z guide for treating many common ailments and illnesses with the help of crystal therapy. It includes a comprehensive colour appendix with photographs and short descriptions of each gemstone recommended.

Michael Gienger
Crystal Massage for Health and Healing
112 Pages, full colour throughout, ISBN 978-1-84409-077-8

This book introduces a spectrum of massage possibilities using healing crystals. The techniques have been developed and refined by experts, and this wisdom is conveyed in simple and direct language, enhanced by photos. Any interested amateur will be amazed at the wealth of new therapeutic possibilities that open up when employing the healing power of crystals.

Michael Gienger, Joachim Goebel
Gem Water
How to prepare and use more than 130 crystal waters for therapeutic treatments
Paperback, 96 pages, ISBN 978-1-84409-131-7

Adding crystals to water is both visually appealing and healthy. It is a known fact that water carries mineral information and Gem Water provides effective remedies, acting quickly on a physical level. It is similar and complementary to wearing crystals, but the effects are not necessarily the same.

Gem Water needs to be prepared and applied with care; this book explains everything you need to know to get started!

Monika Grundmann
Crystal Balance
A step-by-step guide to beauty and health through crystal massage
Paperback, full colour throughout, 112 pages, ISBN 978-1-84409-132-4

Our physical wellbeing reflects every aspect of our lives and inner selves. As a result, massage is able to influence us on every level – mind, body and spirit.

The Crystal Balance method aims to help our bodies relax and recover, encouraging our soul and spirit to 'be themselves'. When we are truly 'ourselves', we are beautiful. It is as simple as that.

Isabel Silveira
Quartz Crystals
A guide to identifying quartz crystals and their healing properties
Paperback, full colour throughout, 80 pages, ISBN 978-1-84409-148-5

This visually impressive book brings the reader up close to the beauty and diversity of the quartz crystal family. Its unique and concise presentation allows the reader to quickly and easily identify an array of quartz crystals and become familiar with their distinctive features and energetic properties.

EARTHDANCER A FINDHORN PRESS IMPRINT

For further information and book catalogue contact:
Findhorn Press, Delft Cottage, Dyke, Forres IV36 2TF, Scotland
Earthdancer Books is an imprint of Findhorn Press.

tel +44 (0)1309-690582   fax +44 (0)131 777 2711
info@findhornpress.com   www.earthdancer.co.uk   www.findhornpress.com

For more information on crystal healing visit www.crystalhealingbooks.com

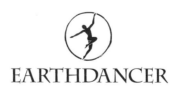

EARTHDANCER

A FINDHORN PRESS IMPRINT